How to lose weight, the easy way!

Una Coales BA (Hons) MD FRCSEd FRCSEd (ENT)
FRCGP DRCOG DFFP PGCertMedEd

www.lulu.com

First published in Great Britain by www.lulu.com 2011.

Published and distributed by Lulu.com
3101 Hillsborough Street,
Raleigh, NC 27607, USA.
Website: www.lulu.com

Copyright © 2011 Dr Una Coales
ISBN 13: 978-1-4478-5865-2

Dr Una Coales asserts the moral right to be
identified as the author of the work.

Conditions of Sale
This book is sold subject to the condition that it shall not, by way of trade or otherwise, be lent, re-sold, hired out or otherwise circulated without the publisher's prior written consent in any form of binding or cover other than that in which it is published and without a similar condition including this condition being imposed on the subsequent purchaser.

I would like to dedicate this book to the late Dr Peter Gooderham MB BChir (1988) MRCGP (1994-2004) LLB (2002) LLM (2004) posthumous PhD (2011) who died unexpectedly at the age of 46 on 9 February 2011 from a fatal heart attack. I wish I had written this book for him sooner.

CONTENTS

Preface   3

Chapter One: How much weight would you like to lose?   8
Pick a number

Chapter Two: Exercise is too much hard work.   14
What's the easiest type of exercise?

Chapter Three: Lifestyle   28

Chapter Four: Calories and Portion Distortion   36

Chapter Five: 'Empty' Calories   46

Chapter Six: Pro-Ana and Pro-Mia websites   50

Chapter Seven: Chromosome 16p11.2 locus   64

Chapter Eight: Childhood Obesity   70

Chapter Nine: The truth behind diet tablets   76

Chapter Ten: Tools of the trade   82

Chapter Eleven: Maintenance   92

Chapter Twelve: 10 reasons not to be obese   96

PREFACE

Now that you have decided you both 'want' and 'need' to lose weight, optimize your chances of not only losing weight but keeping the weight off! No more yo-yo diets or hunger strikes. No more fad diets. No more odd food restrictions. No more signing up to a gym's membership for a year and dropping out within the first month. No more monthly supply of diet tablets over the counter. You will lose weight the natural way, and keep it off!

As a GP, I am asked time and time again, 'how do I lose weight? I don't eat that much doctor.' Patients often come in complaining of back pain, 'tired all the time', or other potentially weight-related problems. And when I relay the news that their body mass index (ratio of weight in kilograms vs. height in metres squared) is now above 30 which means they are now 'clinically obese' and then go on to explain the inherent health and cancer risks that come associated with obesity, they look sullen and hopeless. With my hands bound by the 10-minute NHS consultation I am allowed per patient, how do I even begin to show them how easy it is to lose weight, when I and many other GPs are restricted by the 10 minutes we have allocated per patient?

So I have decided to write a book for the public on how to lose weight. It is so easy! When I presented Channel 4's Turn Back Your Body Clock in 2006 which has now aired globally and is seen as far afield as Dubai and Singapore on BBC Lifestyle Channel, I was privileged to have 8 kind contributors who took part in the television series for 8 weeks of their lives and each lost weight! It was a 100% weight loss success rate and the most that was lost was 4 stone in 8 weeks! I am also happy to show you how it was done.

So whether you have a stubborn 10 lbs to lose before your wedding or 100 lbs to lose to get out of the 'clinically obese' category, or whether you dream of being a size 8 again after slowly creeping up to a dress size 14 or getting back into your skinny jeans or transforming into a hot beach babe, this book will show you how to make a successful transition from 'clinically obese' to 'healthy normal' without even breaking into a sweat, the easy way!

Dr Una Coales BA (Hon) MD FRCSEd FRCSEd (ENT)
FRCGP DRCOG DFFP PGCertMedEd
TV Presenter of Channel 4's Turn Back Your Body Clock,
Portfolio NHS and Media GP, Motivational Speaker,
Private Educator and Prolific Author
www.drunacoales.com
September 2011

CHAPTER ONE: HOW MUCH WEIGHT WOULD YOU LIKE TO LOSE? PICK A NUMBER.

Some of you will know precisely how much weight you would like to lose. Some of you have no idea what your ideal weight should be based on your height and bone structure. If you know how much weight you would like to lose then skip this chapter. For those who haven't a clue, first find someone of your similar build who you would like to look like, body weight-wise. This may mean googling images of celebrities you would like to emulate or asking co-workers for their weight. One well-known iconic figure is Kate, the Duchess of Cambridge. She stirred slight media controversy when pro-Ana (pro-anorexia) websites wished to have her represent their ideal. However if we look at how she lost weight and her change in lifestyle, it is not surprising that she did lose weight. She added exercise, i.e. royal walkabouts to her daily routine. So if you do select Kate as your ideal, add on a few pounds as her body mass index is most likely in the underweight range.

Alternatively, you may use the medical BMI (body mass index) guide. A person of normal weight has a BMI between 19 and 25. Overweight is classified as anywhere between a BMI of 26 and 29 and obese for a BMI of 30 or above. Morbid obesity is reserved for a BMI of 40 or above and comes with risks of sudden death from a fatal heart attack. According to the British Heart Foundation, in the United Kingdom, someone is having a heart attack every 2 minutes!

To use the BMI guide, if you stand 5'2" tall, your height in metric is 1.57 metres. One inch equates to 2.54 centimetres so 62 inches equates to 157.5 centimetres or 1.57 metres. The BMI is calculated as weight (kilograms) divided by height (in metres) squared. So to achieve a BMI of 20 at a height of 1.57 metres, one has to aim for a weight of 49 kilograms.

Practice plugging in your height in metres into the equation, multiplying your height by height, ie 1.57 x 1.57 = 2.46 and then using different weights in kilograms to see what kind of BMI number you get.

Here are a few examples of how to calculate your ideal BMI. Note the BMI chart is the same for men and women! Use the WHO (world health organization) BMI chart for growing teenagers, i.e. those 16 and under.

1. Height 5' 7". What should my ideal weight be?

12 inches x 5 feet = 60 inches.

Add 7 inches to 60 and get 67 inches.

67 inches x 2.54 cms to the inch = 170 cms.

170 cms = 1.7 metres.

1.7 metres x 1.7 metres = 2.89. Remember it is not 1.7 x 2 but height squared or height x height.

If we aim for a BMI of 20, then 2.89 x 20 = 58 kilograms.

There are 2.2 lbs in each kilogram. So 58 kilograms x 2.2 lbs/kg = 127 lbs.

There are 14 lbs in each stone. So 127 lbs divided by 14 lbs/stone = 9 stone and 1 lb.

So the ideal weight for a small framed lady of 5' 7" in height is 9 stone.

If your wrist size is large, i.e. an indication that you are big-boned, then aim for a BMI of 25 or 2.89 x 25 = 72 kilograms = 159 lbs = 11 stone 5 lbs.

2. Height 5' 10". What should my ideal weight be?

12 inches x 5 feet = 60 inches.

Add 10 inches to 60 and get 70 inches.

70 inches x 2.54 cms to the inch = 178 cms.

178 cms = 1.78 metres.

1.78 metres x 1.78 metres = 3.55.

If we aim for a BMI of 20, then 3.55 x 20 = 71 kilograms.

There are 2.2 lbs in each kilogram. So 71 kilograms x 2.2 lbs/kg = 156 lbs.

There are 14 lbs in each stone. So 156 lbs divided by 14 lbs/stone = 11 stone 2 lbs.

So the ideal weight for a small framed lady of 5'10" in height is 11 stone.

If we aim for a BMI of 25, then 3.55 x 25 = 88 kilograms.

There are 2.2 lbs in each kilogram. So 88 kilograms x 2.2 lbs/kg = 193 lbs.

There are 14 lbs in each stone. So 193 lbs divided by 14 lbs/stone = 13 stone 11 lbs.

CHAPTER TWO: EXERCISE IS TOO MUCH HARD WORK! WHAT'S THE EASIEST TYPE OF EXERCISE?

I used to think like that. I tried joining a gym to maintain a healthy lifestyle but only felt demoralized when I attempted to participate in the pilates class. I wasn't even over-weight, yet could not keep up with the pace of the class!

Running on a treadmill was no better. I had no interest in staring at myself in a mirror opposite the treadmill and running on the spot. In fact as a novice at exercise, my exercise tolerance level was so low that I would be out of breath after 4 minutes. So I completely empathize with the majority of you out there who cannot get past this 'exercise' mental block.

I also got short of breath climbing up a flight of stairs in hospital so would often opt for the lift! So if you are like me with no exercise stamina, then believe me if I have found a way to incorporate easy exercise into my lifestyle, so can you!

GPs also face this problem with weight-gain in their 40s as they leave their active hospital-based jobs for the sedentary lifestyle of a GP, sitting at a desk for hours on end.

Have you often asked yourself, how did I fit into a size 8 dress in college, yet now 20 years later, I am a size 14? And often one uses the 'excuse' that metabolism slows down in middle-age. Actually, it is not metabolism but physical activity. In college, one would walk around campus from class to class carrying a backpack full of heavy books. If the lift did not come in time and one was running late for class, one took the stairs. Weekends were often spent dancing the night away. Then as we get older, we take on a job. The job may involve standing in place for 8 hours a day or sitting at a desk for 8 hours a day. Suddenly we have become stationary. So each hour of the day is spent burning fewer calories than if we were back at college, walking from class to class.

I then reflected back at my time doing a surgical residency training programme in New York City. My lowest weight was a mere 87 lbs or 6 stone 3 lbs! I was horrified to see the exposed ribs in my back. Yet I had not been dieting? How did I get so thin? I then had a look at my lifestyle. I had gone from being at medical school, walking to and from class for 8 hours a day to being a surgical trainee working 100 hour a week shifts! Every other day I was working a 36-hour shift from 7 am to 1 pm the next day! I was eating 3 meals a day but during the night shift, the hospital canteen was closed and I was not eating enough for the amount of exercise I was doing, walking from the emergency room, standing in the operating room theatre for hours at night and walking to and from the different wards that spanned the entire hospital, checking in on patients. So what I had inadvertently done was dramatically increase my level of walking and standing activity from 8 hours a day to 36-hour shifts at 100 hours a week and at 250 calories an hour of walking, my body had no choice but to lose weight as I was burning off more than I was able to eat. In fact each week I was burning off up to a whopping 25,000 calories yet only consuming a normal daily maintenance intake of 1,200 calories a day or 8,400 calories a week. Once I realized what had happened, I then had to increase my food intake (fuel) to double the normal amount to regain weight to the normal healthy range.

Is it no wonder that celebrities who enroll in the television series 'Strictly come dancing' lose weight, as ballroom dancing burns 158 calories every 30 minutes or 320 calories every hour of rehearsal! And it is not surprising, that once training stops, some regain weight. This is also seen with some singers who go on tour and perform each night but once the tour is over, they put on weight. What is happening is while on tour, they are actively burning off extra calories, i.e. losing weight without trying, but when they return to their sedentary lifestyle, they continue to eat as much food for less activity, so put on weight.

So there I was, perplexed at how to introduce exercise into my lifestyle when I was always the last to be picked for school teams in physical education when the answer was staring me in the face. It was only when I came across a most fascinating statistic, i.e. walking for 1.5 hours burns off up to 400 calories, i.e. an entire meal! This was an amazing Eureka moment for me. So I didn't have to break out a sweat anymore for an activity to be classified as exercise! Walking WAS exercise! And walking is the EASIEST form of exercise that you and I can do without breaking into a sweat!

This then made it clear why those who unfortunately become morbidly obese have little chance of losing weight once they become confined to a wheel chair or bed. Suddenly all activity has stopped, even the easiest, walking.

Here is something I came across while 'googling' for calories and activities. This is a chart of calories burned for 30 minutes of each type of activity. Have a look and see what type of activity you can and would like to do.

30 minutes of these activities for a 120 lb person, will burn:

GYM ACTIVITIES

Aerobics, low impact: 158
Aerobics, high impact: 202
Aerobics, Step low impact: 202
Aerobics, Step high impact: 288
Aerobics, water: 115
Bicycling, Stationery, moderate: 202
Bicycling, Stationery, vigorous: 302
Calisthenics, vigorous: 230
Calisthenics, moderate: 130
Circuit Training, general: 230
Elliptical Trainer, general: 259
Riders: general: 144

Rowing, Stationery, moderate: 202
Rowing, Stationery, vigorous: 245
Ski Machine general: 274
Stair Step Machine general: 173
Stretching, Yoga: 115
Teaching aerobics: 173
Weight Lifting: general 86
Weight Lifting: vigorous 173

TRAINING AND SPORT ACTIVITIES

Archery: non-hunting 101
Badminton general: 130
Basketball playing a game: 230
Basketball wheelchair: 187
Billiards: 72
Bicycling BMX or mountain: 245
Bicycling 12-13.9 mph: 230
Bicycling 14-15.9 mph: 288
Bicycling 16-19 mph: 346
Bicycling > 20 mph: 475
Bowling: 86
Boxing sparring: 259
Curling: 115
Dancing Fast, ballet, twist: 173
Dancing disco, ballroom, square: 158
Dancing slow, waltz, foxtrot: 86
Fencing: 173
Football competitive: 259
Football touch, flag, general: 230
Frisbee: 86Golf carrying clubs: 158
Golf using cart: 101
Gymnastics general: 115
Handball general: 346
Hang Gliding: 101
Hiking cross-country: 173

Hockey field & ice: 230
Horseback Riding: general 115
Ice Skating general: 202
Kayaking: 144
Martial Arts judo, karate, kickbox: 288
Race Walking: 187
Racquetball competitive: 288
Racquetball casual, general: 202
Rock Climbing ascending: 317
Rock Climbing rapelling: 230
Rollerblade Skating: 202
Rope Jumping: 288
Running 5 mph (12 min/mile): 230
Running 5.2 mph (11.5 min/mile): 259
Running 6 mph (10 min/mile): 288
Running 6.7 mph (9 min/mile): 317
Running 7.5 mph (8 min/mile): 360
Running 8.6 mph (7 min/mile): 418
Running 10 mph (6 min/mile): 475
Running pushing wheelchair, marathon wheeling: 230
Running cross-country: 259
Scuba or skin diving: 202
Skateboarding: 144
Skiing: cross-country: 230
Skiing: downhill: 173
Sledding, luge, toboggan: 202
Snorkeling: 144
Soccer general: 202
Swimming general: 173
Swimming laps, vigorous: 288
Swimming backstroke: 230
Swimming breaststroke: 288
Swimming butterfly: 317
Swimming crawl: 317
Swimming treading, vigorous: 288
Tai Chi: 115

Tennis general: 202
Volleyball non-competitive, general play: 86
Volleyball competitive, gymnasium play: 115
Volleyball beach: 230
Walk 3.5 mph (17 min/mi): 115
Walk 4 mph (15 min/mi): 130
Walk 4.5 mph (13 min/mi): 144
Walk/Jog (jog 10 min): 173
Water Skiing: 173
Water Polo: 288
Water Volleyball: 86
Whitewater (rafting, kayaking): 144
Wrestling 173

OUTDOOR ACTIVITIES

Carrying & stacking wood: 144
Chopping & splitting wood: 173
Digging, spading dirt: 144
Gardening (general): 130
Gardening (weeding): 133
Laying sod / crushed rock:144
Mowing Lawn (push, hand): 158
Mowing Lawn (push, power): 130
Operate Snow Blower (walking): 130
Planting seedlings, shrubs: 115
Plant trees: 130
Raking Lawn: 115
Sacking grass or leaves: 115
Shoveling Snow (by hand): 173

HOME AND DAILY LIFE ACTIVITIES

Child-care (bathing, feeding, etc.): 101
Child games (hop-scotch, jacks, etc.): 144
Cooking: 72

Food Shopping (with cart): 101
Heavy Cleaning (wash car, windows): 130
Moving (household furniture): 173
Moving (carrying boxes): 202
Moving (unpacking): 101
Playing w/kids (moderate effort): 115
Playing w/kids (vigorous effort): 144
Reading: sitting: 32
Standing in line: 36
Sleeping: 18
Watching TV: 22
Home Repair
Auto Repair: 86
Carpentry: (outside) 173
Carpentry: (refinish furniture) 130
Cleaning rain gutters: 144
Hanging storm windows: 144
Lay or remove carpet/tile: 130
Paint house: (outside) 144
Paint, paper, remodel: (inside) 130
Roofing: 173
Wiring and Plumbing: 86

OCCUPATIONAL ACTIVITIES

Bartending/Server: 72
Carpentry Work: 101
Coaching Sports: 115
Coal Mining: 173
Computer Work: 40
Construction, general: 158
Desk Work: 50
Firefighting: 346
Forestry, general: 230
Heavy Equip. Operator: 72
Heavy Tools, not power: 230

Horse Grooming: 173
Light Office Work: 43
Masonry: 202
Masseur, standing: 115
Police Officer: 72
Sitting in Class: 50
Sitting in Meetings: 47
Steel Mill: (general) 230
Theater Work: 86
Truck Driving: sitting 58
Welding: 86

This explains why your teenagers are as thin as rakes and you as a middle-aged parent are struggling to lose weight. Now perusing the list, find the easiest activity that would still classify as exercise. I have highlighted my daily activities. The only difference I made, to try out my own weight loss plan, as advocated by my book, was to add exercise in the form of walking at 17 minutes per mile which burns off 115 calories every 30 minutes or 230 calories an hour. I wouldn't count sitting at work or at meetings at 47 calories per 30 minutes or about 100 calories an hour. So if you want to lose weight faster, opt for the walking activity rather than the sitting method.

Oddly enough the list does not include house work under home activities so award yourself 100 calories every 30 minutes or 200 calories an hour for light housework. You see, I am going for the easy option and still can show you, how you CAN lose weight without breaking a sweat!

'No pain, no gain' is reserved for those extremists who need to lose 4 stone in 8 weeks because 2 million television viewers will be watching you. The television contributor pushed the boundaries of pain by pushing up his cardio exercise when his weight loss reached a plateau. I would only recommend rigorous exercise for those who have a strong heart and prior exercise training experience. But for the majority of us, light regular exercise 4 x 4 is much more manageable.

So mix and match your 4 x 4 of walking. That's 4 hours of walking x 4 days a week and can be a mixture of window shopping, tube travel, grocery shopping, light housework preferably up and down stairs and walking to/from work.

The National Weight Control Registry (www.nwcr.ws) records details of 5,000 people who have lost an average of 66 lbs and kept it off for at least 5.5 years with walking exercise and food modification! Walking IS exercise! Hallelujah we have found a way to lose weight through exercise that does not involve breaking out into a sweat and everyone, young and old can walk!

CHAPTER THREE: LIFESTYLE

Now that we have decided on the easiest form of exercise, how do we incorporate this into our lifestyle so that it becomes habit and we can maintain our weight loss also, i.e. no yo-yo weight gain. To lose weight, I am asking you to fit in 4 hours of walking 3-4 times a week. Remember the simple walking exercise formula 4 x 4! 4 hours x 4 days a week.

So how are you going to fit in 4 hours a day of walking every other day?

Well have a look at your daily and weekly schedule. Are you a stay-at home mother or working 9-5 Monday to Friday? If you are in the former group, then it is easy to incorporate walking into your schedule. You could walk your children to school, walk to the local supermarket, and even get an all-day travel card and take the tube into town and window-shop.

I decided I was 'too shy' to be a gym member, so decided to put this 'walking-exercise' plan into action and bought a one-day 2-zone underground travel card and took the tube into central London rather than drive. I started to notice that when I was driving, I would never see obese people on the street walking. In fact most of the people walking on the pavement were of normal weight. It then dawned on me that obese people were more likely to drive or stay at home. So by making the effort to ditch the car three times a week and take the tube, I was already losing weight as I was changing my lifestyle to incorporate walking!

Did you know that walking from one end of the underground platform to the other end where the exit is, as one invariably boards the train at the wrong end of the platform, is a good 200 steps?! And then I mentally added up the effort it was taking to climb stairs and walk from one end of the station to another to change lines. In fact Green Park tube station is the best for exercise as it is the longest walk to change from the Victoria to the Piccadilly line! So return travel by tube was already burning off an hour of walking exercise!

This then can be incorporated into the lifestyle of those who work. Leave your car at home and take the tube or British Rail. To lose weight drastically, try walking home from work instead of taking the tube! One investment banker ditched the Northern line and walked home from the City every evening, lost 2 stone and looked 10 years younger as an added bonus! Once you have made the lifestyle change permanent, you know you will not rebound and regain the weight at the end of the book.

If you are struggling to find 4 hours a day of walking exercise, take the stairs at work, take advantage of late-night shopping hours, spend the entire day out in shopping malls on weekends or take an excursion by coach to a premium designer outlet mall.

If you are a GP, then cycle to home visits. If you are or are not a GP, then cycle to work.

Be creative as to how to incorporate walking 4 hours a day every other day into your weekly lifestyle.

To give myself an incentive to walk for 4 x 4 a week (4 hours x 4 days a week), I purchased a 2-zone all day London transport travel card and took the tube and bus to the high street. In 4 hours I could cover Oxford Street, Bond Street, Knightsbridge and King's Road with a combination of walking and public transport. The incentive was to go 'bargain-hunting' for a new modern wardrobe. I, like many women of my age, get stuck wearing clothes of a certain bygone era. To fund these walking/shopping excursions, I thinned out my wardrobe and listed most of my clothing on ebay. Suddenly my walking exercise became fun!

Remember daily housework for 30 minutes a day also counts as walking exercise. So do a bit of housework (cleaning surfaces, hoovering, making beds, doing laundry) every morning before work to kick start your metabolism at an energy expenditure of 100 calories an hour.

If you have a teenager who needs to lose weight, then get her a free bus pass for under 16s. Have her enjoy the freedom of travelling on the bus with school friends and walking up and down Kings Road.

A more drastic way to lose weight is to also reduce the hours of inactivity, so limiting the hours spent in front of a computer or television screen. Yes, I called it drastic as we are all addicted to watching our favourite sitcom or news channel and of course social networking has become a sedentary habit-forming past-time or dare I say addiction!

It comes as no surprise that even our children are at risk of obesity these days with the advent of the 42-inch plasma television screens and the price reduction from £3,000 to £500 so that most families can now afford and own a super-sized plasma television. And now family-life seems to be centred around the television instead of a traditional fireplace hearth. Make it a rule to at least turn off the television during family meals!

You have completed chapter three once you have finally worked out how to incorporate 4 hours of walking every other day into your weekly schedule so that it becomes a life-long habit. You see how many times I have repeated the phrase 'incorporate 4 hours of walking'! So now do it! And if you are still finding excuses, pull out a picture of your favourite celebrity or a size 8 dress to remind yourself why you desperately want to lose weight and will!

CHAPTER FOUR: CALORIES AND PORTION DISTORTION

Calories are a unit of energy. One often hears of 'calories in' has to equal 'calories out'. An analogy used is fuel for a car. Food is the fuel needed to run a car. What if we supply too much fuel to our car? Well the good news is that one cannot physically pour more fuel than the container holds. Unfortunately human beings are not exactly cars and we can keep pouring fuel into our bodies as the stomach just expands. The danger is the more it expands, the more we need to eat to feel the 'full' sensation.

There are 24 million overweight people in the UK of which up to 13 million are obese (BMI > 30). There are over 1 billion overweight people in the world of which 300 million are obese according to the World Health Organisation.

Obesity is set to cost the NHS more than £6 billion a year by 2015 according to Professor Haslam.

The US is the leading country when it comes to world obesity. Australia is second and the UK third. So how did we as a Western World get so fat?

The National Heart Lung and Blood Institute Obesity Education Initiative have coined the phrase Portion Distortion. Did you know that dinner plate sizes have almost doubled in 20 years?

http://hp2010.nhlbihin.net/oei_ss/PD1/download/pdf/PDI.pdf

http://hp2010.nhlbihin.net/oei_ss/PDII/download/pdf/PD2.pdf

In these 2 PDF files you can watch a slide show of how portion sizes have drastically doubled in size as compared with over 20 years ago. Here they also add that 2.5 hours of housework burns of 560 calories. Nice to know!

One of the slides depicts a normal 8 oz cup of coffee at 45 calories compared with a modern day 16 oz mocha coffee at.....a whopping 350 calories! And how can this be you ask? Think full-fat milk and chocolate! That's how! And 200 calorie muffins used to be normal sized but have now been superseded by large muffins at 500-700 calories, depending on what you have in the muffin as extra! And if you think you can eat salads and lose weight, think again. A chicken Caesar salad in restaurants is a whopping 790 calories! In other words, you are consuming extra 'hidden' calories without even being aware. A popcorn box at the cinema has 630 calories, that's almost 2 meals!

What does that tell you? It tells you that the Western consumerist world is trying to make you consume more food and drink? Is it no wonder that in third world countries, devoid of cars and public transportation and ready-made meals and fast food drive-through restaurants, that the population is normal or underweight?

So how can we decide on what to eat if everything out there has been super-sized to create a super-sized morbidly obese population? Are we to go from a nation of 2-legged bi-pedals to a nation of couch potatoes and beached whales? Sorry to be so blunt but we do have to come to the realisation that this is happening all around us and how to stop this.

I said 'the easy way' so here goes. This chapter ends with a list of meals you may eat as breakfast, lunch or dinner, feel full and still lose weight. The key is to find meals in the 200-300 calorie range and stick to a 900 calories a day intake while losing weight. The choices on the list both make you feel full and 'I can't believe it is only 200-300 calories!'

This is why products like Weight Watchers based on points rather than calories are successful but this must be used in combination with exercise (my suggestion is walking) and a permanent change to one's lifestyle so that the weight does not rebound.

Alternatively you may wish to purchase the paperback book Calorie King, Calorie Fat and Carbohydrate Counter with its free website of support www.calorieking.com. I love this book as it lists calories for every fast food restaurant and ready meal out there! There is no escape or denying that you have just consumed a 205 calorie Krispy Kreme donut or a 530 calorie tall Strawberries and Cream from Starbucks. This weight loss plan is not about starvation so if you crave your favourite frappucino from Starbucks then make sure you share it with a friend or even better 2 friends, so you end up consuming only 1/3 of the total calories. Every popular restaurant is listed in the book with their entire calorie-counted menu!

Get in the habit of eating one-course meals. Why has it become a habit to eat three-course meals?

Here is a sample list of meals in the 200-300 calorie range to mix and match while on your weight-reduction plan or to incorporate into your lifestyle to make a permanent change. Remember eat regular meals, 3 times a day and no snacking! Your body must not think it is going into starvation mode or your metabolism will shut down.

So if you are out and about, before you decide on your meal, check first as to whether you are consuming hidden extra whopping calories!

BREAKFAST MENU (SELECT ONE)

Oatmeal with semi skimmed milk (145-200 calories)

English breakfast with 1 small pork sausage, 1 toast, and 1 fried egg (300 calories). You may substitute any for mushrooms and tomatoes.

Instant breakfast cereals (Special K, Frosties) 110-120 calories per cup.

Fresh fruit cups (70 calories per 4 oz size). Double or triple up if eating as a meal.

LUNCH OR DINNER MENU (SELECT ONE)

Broiled lean sirloin steak, medium 5 oz size (265 calories)

Cooked spaghetti, medium size (185 calories)

Heinz Big Soup (the Beef Stew range contains beef, potatoes and vegetables and is only 200 calories for the entire can!)

Japanese Udon noodles (250 calories)

Lamb chop, lean, roasted (155 calories) versus broiled (85 calories) with mashed potato (120 calories) versus baked potato with grated cheese (370 calories)

McDonalds Medium McChicken sandwich (370 calories) – not healthy but if you have an insatiable craving for McDonalds...remember this diet is not about restricting foods just calories and quantity.

Omelette, 2 eggs with cheese (360 calories)

Pret a Manger deluxe sushi box (365 calories)

Pret a Manger tuna salad bowl (370 calories)

Roast beef, 3-4 lean slices (245 calories)

Wagamama chicken mandarin salad (350 calories) versus Chicken katsu curry (800 calories)

Wagamama mini cha-han (200 calories) with miso soup versus Chicken cha han (478 calories)

Wagamama yaki udon (350 calories) versus Chili beef ramen (911 calories!)

Feel free to go through the Calorie King paperback book and add to your list of appetite-satiating, tummy-filling meals in the 200-300 calorie range. You'll be surprised by what you can eat in this range and experience the 'I can't believe it is only 200 calories!' reaction. It is a matter of incorporating these meals into your daily routine for life. Make it a habit of choosing the meal which is both tasty, filling and yet only 200-300 calories! Don't let those hidden extra calories in meals you had no idea had 900 calories sabotage your goal of a hot beach body!

There is a global move towards putting calorie content on food wrappers in McDonalds, on wall menu charts in Starbucks, and hopefully one day, all restaurants will list calorie content next to the prices of each meal, so that you are not inadvertently led to consume 'extra hidden' calories and gain weight exponentially but have the freedom and awareness to choose the option that fulfills your appetite with a normal amount of calories. The food industry is making us fat! They must assume some responsibility for super-sizing and super-calorie adding meals!

CHAPTER FIVE: EMPTY CALORIES

This term I apply to all the drinks we consume which contain 'empty' calories that don't fill us up as a meal does but does end up on our tummy, rear and thighs as unwanted lumps and bumps. So while applying this weight reduction programme, let's ensure we only drink still water which has zero added calories.

During the Turn Back Your Body Series, contributors promised to drink water and abstain from alcohol (a known appetite stimulant) for 8 weeks. They exercised up to 6 times a week. If you are after drastic extreme and fast weight loss, then increase your walking exercise from 3-4 times a week to 6 times a week for 4-5 hours. The male contributor who lost 4 stone in 8 weeks worked out 6 days a week for 6 hours a day mostly running on a treadmill. The banker who lost 2 stone in a month walked for an hour a day 5 times a week and worked out on a treadmill once a week. Both men burned off excessive amounts of calories at an alarming rate by doubling up on the exercise (walking or use of treadmill).

So here is a sample of the drinks to consider avoiding while we are losing weight and even to consider avoiding in the long-term, switching to the diet sugar-free versions or limiting:

Canned soft drinks with sugar

Coca Cola (140 calories)

Pepsi (165 calories)

Fanta (180 calories)

7-Up (140 calories)

Energy drinks with sugar

Gatorade (50 calories)

original Lucozade (350 calories)

Red Bull (113 calories)

Alcoholic beverages (7 calories per gram)

Beer (150 calories)

Champagne (85 calories)

Mai Tai (220 calories)

Red or white wine (80-90 calories)

If you are out with your mates, then either stick to diet sodas or alternate with water in between drinks. Try sipping your wine and taking an hour to finish a glass so that you are seen with a glass in your hand but no need to keep asking for seconds.

However be wary as alcohol is an appetite stimulant and will make you voraciously hungry! Beer used to be served to NHS patients who suffered from anorexia due to cancer. So why would you consume an appetite stimulant if you are trying to lose weight?

You may drink tea or coffee as it is often a morning habit for many. Just top up with semi-skimmed milk. Drinking a cup of filtered freshly brewed coffee can speed up your metabolism also.

Think water and plenty of it to clean out your system and hydrate your cells! Works wonders for a youthful fresh complexion also.

CHAPTER SIX: PRO-ANA AND PRO-MIA WEBSITES

Some of you, especially younger vulnerable women, may be drawn to exploring the world of pro-Ana (pro-anorexia) and pro-Mia (pro-bulimia) websites. Be very wary as what these sites are doing is creating a false sense of belonging and acceptance targeting women who see controlling food intake as a means of dealing with external stressors.

Often times women drawn into anorexia or bulimia suffer from lack of control in their home environment or dare I say lack of love. The sound of a verbally abusive parent may easily become a trigger for a young girl to starve herself. 'I just want my dad to stop shouting at me?' One reads on these sites. What is happening is that young girls find themselves responding much like a Pavlovian dog response of salivation to the sound of a bell trigger. This is a form of

Skinnerian operand conditioning. Or simply put a young girl finds herself experiencing loss of appetite triggered by an abusive parent. Eating disorder sufferers often have a history of childhood abuse (physical, mental and/or sexual). And it is no surprise that family counselling has been proven to be the most effective intervention as an alternative to the $30,000 a month in-patient rehabilitation centres.

There are two nuclei in our brain. The ventro-medial nucleus (VMN) is the satiety nucleus in the hypothalamus which tells us we are full and the lateral hypothalamic nucleus which tells us we are hungry. Ana teens turn on the VMN satiety nucleus and turn off the lateral hypothalamic hunger nucleus by food aversion operant conditioning, by reinforcing hunger strikes with social networks and blogs and by strong pro ana visual images/stimuli. They build friendships with other teens based on how much they lose, i.e. associate weight loss with positive social belonging.

In-patient hospital interventions include intravenous fluid hydration, gastrostomy (stomach tube) feeds, and cognitive behavioural therapy to change thoughts and behaviours. Teens may find themselves isolated from families except for the counseling sessions where they are brought together.

Ana teens often say 'the only thing I am good at is losing weight.' This is a sad yet revealing confession. If you are a parent of an Ana teen, try to boost their self-confidence by finding another 'thing' they can be good at...singing, dancing, art, music, baton swirling, anything but self-starvation.

A solution for Anas would be to change the trigger and association. Better to teach abusive parents to reward eating with hugs and kisses. Parental love = food. But be careful that we stop this association when the teen has reached normal weight or it could swing the other way and the teen finds themselves over-eating to receive more love and attention.

One Ana teen explained that once she went on a sunny holiday with her mother, a switch turned on, and she was hungry again and ate normally. She was cured.

To switch off the lateral hypothalamus hunger nucleus, Anas preoccupy their minds with mindless activity, writing up their social blogs, obsessive exercise for 5 hours a day, 1500 steps in their hospital room, 1000 daily push-ups, 1000 daily sit ups in other words adopt a version of obsessive-compulsive personality disorder.

Ana teens are often between 10 and 14 years of age, so do not drink alcohol which turns on the lateral hypothalamus nucleus for hunger, which accounts for why most middle- aged people are overweight. Their hunger nucleus is almost always on with alcohol intake and stays on for 24 hours after consumption.

On my show 'Turn Back Your Body Clock', we used visual imagery, i.e. 3-dimensional magnetic resonance images of a contributor's obese body to force the contributor to be upfront about his or her obesity and not hide in denial. Strong lines like 'Your body is completely encased in fat!' were used to drive home the point that obesity was not acceptable and that to treat one's body in this manner was a form of self-harm and abuse. Often times an obese person will not look in a mirror or even own a full-length mirror. With this both profound and personal visual imagery, we had temporarily turned off the lateral hypothalamus hunger nucleus or simply put, made the contributor think twice before consuming large quantities of food and made him or her reflect on the damage over-eating could and had caused.

Blood tests with high cholesterol, blood pressures showing high blood pressure and liver scans showing fatty liver also drove home the message that obesity causes serious health problems and an early death. This was always countered with hope, the good news that we could fix this and reverse the damage, and we succeeded with a joint effort between the television production team and the contributors.

Interestingly when the television crew and I settled to a pub lunch, the contributor declined to join us and said he would make himself a healthy lunch at home! He had changed his lifestyle and already adopted healthy eating. It had become a life-forming habit!

What is happening to the majority of the population, both working and unemployed? Why are they struggling to lose weight? Well let us contrast their habits with that of pro-anas (the weight-loss extremist). Obese people are often inactive and sit at their computers or watch television or doing both watching television on one's own computer on BBC iplayer! What comes on the television? Food commercials, food and cooking imagery in shows like 'Come dine with me', 'Gordon Ramsay's kitchen nightmares', etc. And often times if there is a television movie, the characters are filmed eating at a restaurant. So inadvertently by watching too much television, the public are getting subliminal images to suggest they eat all the time!

If one were at a job where there was no on-site canteen, but just the job at hand to preoccupy one's mind, one is more inclined to lose weight. So if you must watch television, select shows where eating and drinking do not feature so heavily! How about 'Escape to the Country', 'Nothing to Declare', 'X-factor' or 'Antique Road Show' perhaps?

Have you ever found an obese teetotaler? I say again drinking alcohol switches on your lateral hypothalamus nucleus in your brain and triggers massive hunger pangs!!! Ever notice how alcohol comes paired with food....beer and pizza, beer and kebab, champagne and canapes, etc.

If you have a loved one who needs to lose weight for health reasons, do him or her a kindness and bin the alcohol!

And if your loved one needs 'alcohol aversion therapy', have him select from the list below:

1. Visit a patient on a head and neck ward or any cancer ward and sit down and chat with a real person suffering from throat cancer. Alcohol is associated with throat cancer!

2. Visit your local hospice and sit down with a terminal cancer-sufferer.

3. Ask around and see who among your acquaintances has obtained a driving under the influence conviction and hear how they travelled by bus for a year.

4. Pop into your local hospital emergency room on weekends and see doctors busy suturing lacerations on those involved in drunkard brawls.

5. Volunteer at a local homeless men's hostel and see men with dual diagnoses of alcoholism and mental disease and listen to these forgotten men explain how they once were a famous football goalie, an Asian father who lost his wife, family and job, and how they ended up penniless, homeless and alone.

6. Watch the infamous and sad you-tube clip of David Hasselhoff, in a drunken stupor filmed by his daughter, eating a burger off the loo floor.

Anas rely on over the counter pharmaceuticals to lose weight. Please do not buy diet tablets over the counter, which often contain caffeine or amphetamine-like substances.

Please do not buy over the counter laxatives which can lead to a dangerous drop in your potassium levels. Your body needs this chemical for its muscle and nerve activity. You obtain this naturally from fruit (bananas, strawberries, oranges), meat (beef, turkey, fish) and vegetable (mushrooms). Low potassium can lead to dangerous heart arrhythmias and death.

Pro-ana websites contain and rely on a heavy dose of visual imagery/ stimuli of thin ladies, models, teens, etc. to inspire and keep anorexic girls motivated to continue extreme self-destructive weight loss and encourages girls to browse the photos to keep motivated and stave off hunger pangs, to get through 'the hour'. Often the sight of exposed ribs or vertebrae excites these bloggers!

Having said all this, how can we learn from these sites when tackling the big picture of world obesity which has become an epidemic. The techniques Anas are using are food aversion stimuli coupled with strong imagery to reinforce compliance and motivation and a network of support through blogging.

Looking at these techniques, perhaps we can learn and adopt some of these techniques but in a positive light. Let us try to create a stimulus or a positive association for exercise, a healthy incentive for walking.

Most women enjoy shopping but can't afford to go shopping every day or would go bankrupt! So how about incorporating 'window browsing' as a form of 'walking exercise'. An incentive would be to 'bargain hunt' or trawl the sales racks. Surprisingly sales are still found even in the months of August and September! No longer are sale months confined to July and December. With this global recession, retailers are forever advertising sales! Even if it means walking up and down, in and out of stores in an outlet mall, do it, as it counts as exercise! Your young teenagers do it with friends and stay slim, so too can you!

Strong imagery to reinforce compliance and motivation is an interesting concept. Instead of strong imagery of thinness, how about strong imagery of healthy people enjoying healthy activities and holidays in the sunshine. Fish out your old photo albums and remind yourself of holidays spent when you were of normal weight or of your own wedding. Can you fit back into your wedding dress? Have your wedding dress dry-cleaned and remember the good times when you were not hanging over your seat as your rear was too big for public transport. Remember how easy it was to go into a shop and try on clothes without being embarrassed about asking for a size larger. It is about motivating yourself and finding within yourself a happy time when you were of normal weight and size.

CHAPTER SEVEN: CHROMOSOME 16p11.2 LOCUS

'But doctor, it's in the genes.' Some patients believe that because they come from a 'large' family, they have no hope of losing weight and that no matter how 'little' they eat, they keep gaining weight.

So I looked at two teenagers, aged 13 and 16, who had body mass indexes (BMIs) of approximately 15 and 16, respectively. Based on numbers alone, this would put them both in the 'anorexic' category with a BMI under 17.5. One stands 5'3" in height and weighs a mere 40 kilograms and another 5'8" in stature and weighs only 50 kilograms. I then examined their daily intake (calories in, fuel or energy intake). A typical menu was 2 large waffles with whipped cream and fresh strawberries (at least 500 calories) for breakfast, a Pret-a-Manger duck wrap for lunch (approximately 400 calories) and home-cooked toad in the hole with salad for dinner (500 calories) to add up to a total daily consumption of 1400 calories. This was not a self-starvation diet of 300 calories a day and nor were they resorting to purging or using over the counter pharmaceuticals, so how did they get so thin?

I then asked about their school activities. They walked up and down hills to their classrooms carrying heavy book bags, did evening classes of ballet twice a week, and participated in daily physical education (track and field, tennis or whatever that school term's sport was). So apart from the extra activity of ballet twice a week, they had the same amount of physical activity as all the other students, who by the way, were also on the slender side. By adding up all their physical activity, it was clear that gradually they were burning off more calories (energy out) than they were consuming (energy/fuel in).

Were they weak or tired all the time? Were they pale and anaemic? Did they have electrolyte imbalances? Did they stop menstruating? Did they have fine lanugo (baby) hair? The answer was no. They were both physically very strong and able to lift almost their own body weight! So was it in their family genes to be so slim and yet lead a healthy lifestyle with normal diet and regular exercise?

On August 31, 2011, a research study was published in a scientific journal 'Nature' of how DNA of over 95,000 people identified that duplication of a part of chromosome 16 was associated with extreme thinness, i.e. a BMI of below 18.5. The frequency of this double gene dosage was 1 in 2000 people with men being 23 times and women being 5 times more likely to have this 'defect' and be extremely underweight.

The paper is entitled '*Mirror extreme BMI phenotypes associated with gene dosage at the chromosome 16p11.2 locus.*' Conversely the same researchers discovered that those found to have a deletion of this part of chromosome 16 were 43 times more likely to be morbidly obese.

Professor Philippe Froguel from the School of Public Health at Imperial College, London, led the study and states that, "It's also the first example of a deletion and a duplication of one part of the genome having opposite effects. At the moment we don't know anything about the genes in this region. If we can work out why gene duplication in this region causes thinness, it might throw up new potential treatments for obesity and appetite disorders. We now plan to sequence these genes and find out what they do, so we can get an idea of which ones are involved in regulating appetite."

So does this mean that if you are morbidly obese, you stand no chance of losing weight as it is in your genetic make-up to be extremely obese? Or can environment and external factors overcome what genetics has given us to begin life with?

I say one can overcome nature's inheritance, however it will need more attention to calories in versus calories out. In other words, knowing that your metabolism is slower than the normal adult, means one may have to do more walking to lose the same amount of weight.

One of the contributors on Turn Back Your Body Clock suffered from hypothyroidism. An underactive thyroid is often used as an excuse for gaining weight and not being able to lose the weight due to a slowed metabolism. However even he was able to lose weight on the series! Nurture can overcome Nature!

CHAPTER EIGHT: CHILDHOOD OBESITY

On 13 September 2011, one of the main articles in the London Evening Standard newspaper was one covering childhood obesity. The headline was 'Free meals for primary pupils in obesity fight,' and details how £8 million will be spent over the next three years to offer every primary school pupil in Southwark, South London, a free nutritious lunch each day, regardless of family income. The scheme launched for Reception and Year One students and is due to be rolled out to all 21,000 students across 70 schools as NHS figures show that Southwark has one of the highest levels of childhood obesity in the nation! Childhood obesity costs £7.1 million a year to treat in the London capital.

I would suggest that we also examine 'nurture'. What happens when the child wakes up in the morning? What constitutes breakfast? If the breakfast size and caloric content are excessive, then one nutritious meal amidst two other unhealthy meals with extra hidden calories will not do much to lower the overall total daily intake of calories. What happens when a parent picks up a school child? Does he or she have sweets waiting, a bag of crisps and chocolate bar? How much does the child snack between meals? How large are the portions for dinner? Child-size or adult-size? What does the child drink? Is he or she being given sugary drinks with empty calories enough to constitute an entire meal in calories alone?

And what happened to balancing the equation with exercise? In the United Kingdom, physical education is compulsory in state schools up until the age of 16. What happens next? Well you can guess as well as I can, that once regular exercise at school stops, the weight starts piling on. It can only get worse if a college student living away from home then relies on cheap, fattening convenience foods rather than nutritious home cooking. And before long, a college student who is not a part of a school athletic team, can find him or herself obese on pizza, beer, fish and chips, Indian take-aways, kebabs, Mcdonalds, Burger King, Kentucky Fried Chicken and ready-made meals.

Why are state school students more likely to be obese than public (private) school students? Interestingly, in a private school, the emphasis is on joining a school sports team. So not only do private day or boarding students have their regular quota of scheduled PE (physical education), but they are also invited to explore any talent in fencing, lacrosse, tennis, swimming, gymnastics and so on. In fact, it is highly encouraged as part of presenting a well-rounded student for application to university. Also rota'd in is the Duke of Edinburgh grueling hike with outdoor camping.

Private students mostly come from wealthy families who rely less on instant ready-made meals and fast-food convenience restaurants and more on nutritious home-cooking and fine-food restaurant cuisine. Nurture has a big influence on maintaining normal weight with a normal healthy diet and regular exercise. One is less inclined to hear of a family sitting around the television but more of a family going skiing.

So is childhood obesity resigned to the lower socio-economic classes? Are we building up a stereotype that will adversely affect their job prospects in future also?

Perhaps family education and primary prevention of childhood obesity are more cost-effective than the state paying for weight-loss camps for obese children and paying for free school lunches. Will one free nutritious school lunch a day make much difference if there is a bag of crisps, a bar of chocolate and bag of haribos hiding in their school bag?

CHAPTER NINE: THE TRUTH BEHIND DIET TABLETS

Losing weight should not cost £40 for a monthly supply of over the counter Alli tablets. According to the National Institute of Clinical Excellence report on obesity, GPs may now prescribe the generic version 'orlistat' on a FP 10 prescription for £7.40 to those patients whose body mass index is greater than 30. What is Alli or orlistat? It is the only weight-reduction tablet available on prescription and works by reducing fat absorption. The side-effect is diarrhoea. Some patients have worked out that if they do not take it before a wedding or event requiring large consumptions of cake and fatty foods, they will not get diarrhoea. This however defeats the purpose of this pill to aid in 'teaching' patients which foods will provoke this unwanted side effect and which foods are free or low in fat. Is this the answer?

I say it is better to follow my book and learn how to lose weight the easy way, the cost-free way, the permanent way through simply understanding how one gains and loses weight from calorie intake and calorie expenditure, energy in must equal energy out. There is no need to rely on diet tablets.

Prior to 2010, GPs were also allowed to prescribe sibutramine which was called reductil over the counter. How did this weight-reduction pill work? Well it worked on the brain! The scientific explanation is that it was a centrally-acting serotonin-norepinephrine reuptake inhibitor structurally related to amphetamines! And there in the fine print, we see that patients were actually taking a drug related to amphetamines or speed! It was found to be associated with increased heart attacks and strokes and has been withdrawn from the market in Australia, Canada, China, the European Union (EU), Hong Kong, India, Mexico, Thailand, the UK, and the United States. How many people struggling to lose weight ended up suffering a heart attack or stroke?!

Prior to 2009, GPs were also allowed to prescribe rimonabant, another weight-reducing pill hailed by the pharmaceutical companies as yet another 'cure' or 'wonder drug' combating obesity. Rimonabant was also called SR141716, Acomplia, Bethin, Monaslim, Remonabent, Riobant, Slimona, Rimoslim, Zimulti, and Riomont. It also acted on the brain as a mind-altering drug. In scientific language, it was a selective cannaboid (CB1) receptor blocker in the brain and worked by appetite suppression.

It was made available in the United Kingdom in 2006 and by 2008, was available in 56 countries. However in June 2007, concerns arose over reported side-effects of suicidality and depression associated with use of the drug, and the US Food and Drug Administration were duly made aware.

On 23 October 2008, the European Medicines Agency (EMEA) issued a press release stating its Committee for Medical Products for Human Use (CHMP) had concluded the benefits of Acomplia (rimonabant) no longer out-weighed its risks, and subsequently recommended removal of this product from the UK market. Sanofi-Aventis complied. This drug was officially withdrawn by the EMEA on 16 January 2009. How many people struggling to lose weight took rimonabant and ended up committing suicide as a side-effect?

What pharmaceutical companies do not tell you is that you have your own natural diet tablet! Your body produces two hormones, ghrelin (appetite stimulant) and peptide YY (appetite suppressant). When you do at least one hour of aerobic exercise (i.e. just walk), you increase peptide YY (your natural diet tablet) and decrease ghrelin levels in your body! Hey presto, you eat less, as you are full faster and no more craving to snack! It works and the effects are sustained!

Obesity is a world-wide epidemic and obese people WANT to lose weight. They seek answers in over-the-counter amphetamine or caffeine-containing pills, prescription weight-reducing tablets, herbal remedies, diet plans such as the Atkins low carbohydrate, high protein diet, Jenny Craig's diet food delivery plans and/or costly Weight Watcher memberships. What are all these commercial products missing? The answer is simple education about the easy and natural way to lose weight; the fact that your body secretes its own natural diet tablet through just one hour of aerobic exercise. Walking, food modification and using your own natural diet tablet hormone is a cost-free way to lose weight, and I say it again, the only permanent way to lose weight and keep it off! No more yo-yo diets! No more hunger pangs, starvation, fasting or food strikes! No more bizarre diet fads and avoiding carbohydrates. No more expensive health farms. No more monthly subscriptions to weight loss sites. Education and understanding how your body gains and loses weight is free and permanent.

CHAPTER TEN: TOOLS OF THE TRADE

In summary we now have a target number picked for our ideal weight, a gentle exercise plan of walking 4 x 4 or 4 hours x 4 times a week using a combination of light housework and gentle walking and a 3-meal eating plan of a total of approximately 900 calories a day covering breakfast, lunch and dinner. So let's see what else you need?

Firstly, purchase or borrow a tape measure. This is very important as weight fluctuates with water retention and time of month, so a tape measure can provide more accurate indications that you are indeed losing weight! Hard to spot any difference on a day-to-day basis, but numbers tell the truth! What better incentive than to see your tape measure go from a 28-inch waist to a 27-inch waist to a 26-inch waist?

Tape Measure

With your tape measure record the following and log on a daily or alternate daily basis:

Both biceps circumference (that's the fattest part of your upper arms, including around your 'bat wings')

Chest circumference (bust size)

Waist circumference (thinnest part around your torso and not where your trouser or skirt hang)

Hip circumference (fattest part around your buttocks)

Both thigh circumferences (the fattest parts around your 'thunder thighs')

I don't mince words. I too have flapped my 'bat wings' so relate to all these colloquial terms!

Record in your diary in inches or centimetres, whichever unit is most familiar to you.

What you will notice on a weekly basis, are the inches coming off all limbs and torso! This will be your visual incentive that my plan works and you are losing weight without even breaking into a sweat or feeling hungry!

Weighing scales

Secondly, purchase or borrow a set of bathroom scales. As long as you remember to weigh yourself every 2-3 days, it is okay if you forget to climb on the scales at roughly the same time every morning.

Now a fun modern way to record your weight is on a body mass index (BMI) app. If you own an ipad or iphone, here is a typical entry on a body mass index app.

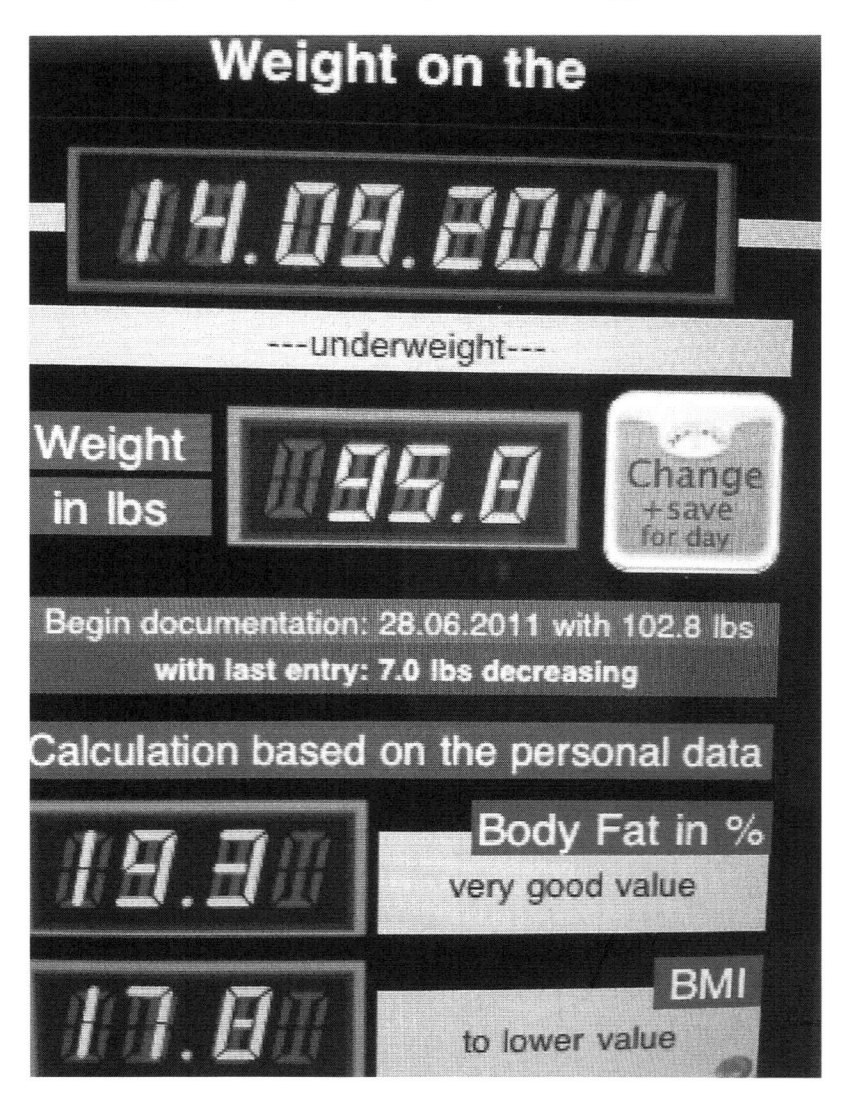

Here are the daily entries that this BMI app allows you to chart your daily, weekly and monthly weight loss progression.

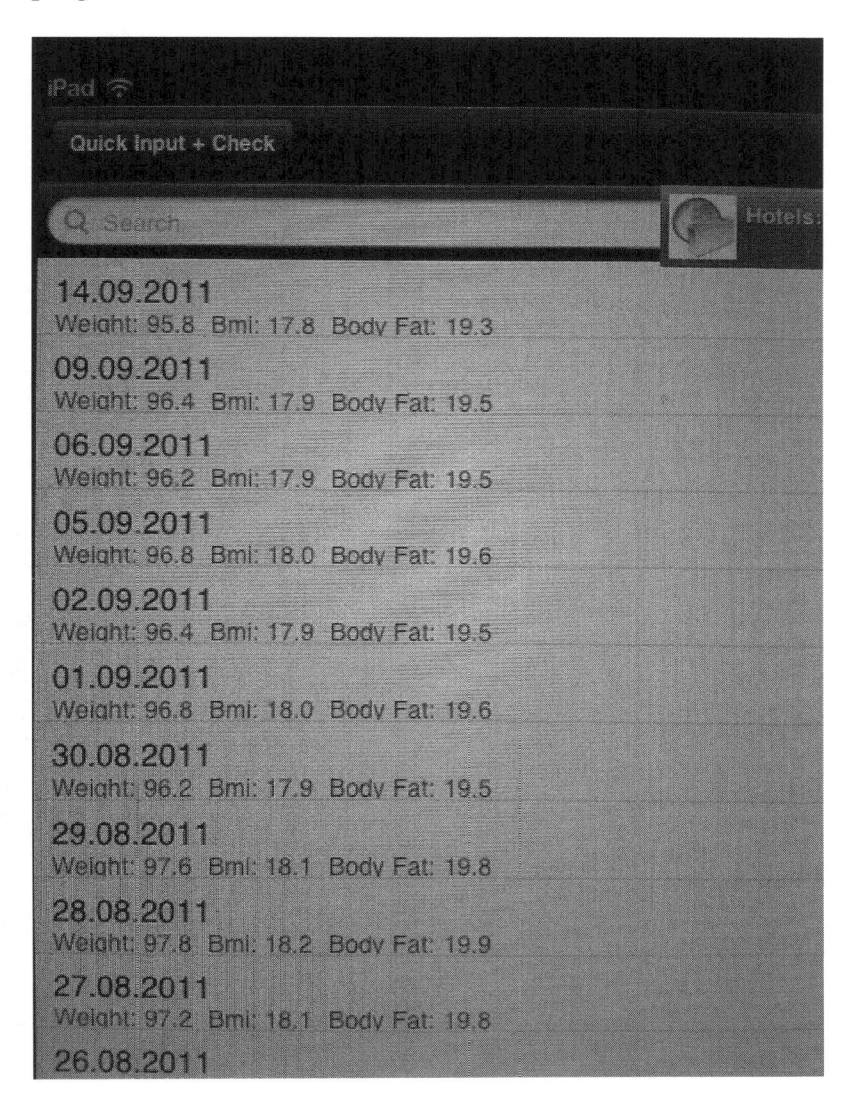

```
iPad
Quick Input + Check
Q Search                                    Hotels

14.09.2011
Weight: 95.8  Bmi: 17.8  Body Fat: 19.3
09.09.2011
Weight: 96.4  Bmi: 17.9  Body Fat: 19.5
06.09.2011
Weight: 96.2  Bmi: 17.9  Body Fat: 19.5
05.09.2011
Weight: 96.8  Bmi: 18.0  Body Fat: 19.6
02.09.2011
Weight: 96.4  Bmi: 17.9  Body Fat: 19.5
01.09.2011
Weight: 96.8  Bmi: 18.0  Body Fat: 19.6
30.08.2011
Weight: 96.2  Bmi: 17.9  Body Fat: 19.5
29.08.2011
Weight: 97.6  Bmi: 18.1  Body Fat: 19.8
28.08.2011
Weight: 97.8  Bmi: 18.2  Body Fat: 19.9
27.08.2011
Weight: 97.2  Bmi: 18.1  Body Fat: 19.8
26.08.2011
```

26.08.2011
Weight: 97.8 Bmi: 18.2 Body Fat: 19.9

25.08.2011
Weight: 96.0 Bmi: 17.8 Body Fat: 19.3

24.08.2011
Weight: 98.2 Bmi: 18.3 Body Fat: 20.1

23.08.2011
Weight: 98.8 Bmi: 18.4 Body Fat: 20.2

21.08.2011
Weight: 98.8 Bmi: 18.4 Body Fat: 20.2

20.08.2011
Weight: 99.4 Bmi: 18.5 Body Fat: 20.4

17.08.2011
Weight: 99.6 Bmi: 18.5 Body Fat: 20.4

16.08.2011
Weight: 99.4 Bmi: 18.5 Body Fat: 20.4

15.08.2011
Weight: 100.4 Bmi: 18.7 Body Fat: 20.7

13.08.2011
Weight: 99.8 Bmi: 18.6 Body Fat: 20.5

11.08.2011
Weight: 99.8 Bmi: 18.6 Body Fat: 20.5

09.08.2011
Weight: 98.8 Bmi: 18.4 Body Fat: 20.2

06.08.2011
Weight: 100.0 Bmi: 18.6 Body Fat: 20.5

05.08.2011

Quick Input + Check

05.08.2011
Weight: 99.8 Bmi: 18.6 Body Fat: 20.5

04.08.2011
Weight: 100.8 Bmi: 18.7 Body Fat: 20.7

03.08.2011
Weight: 101.0 Bmi: 18.8 Body Fat: 20.8

02.08.2011
Weight: 100.8 Bmi: 18.7 Body Fat: 20.7

01.08.2011
Weight: 101.4 Bmi: 18.8 Body Fat: 20.8

30.07.2011
Weight: 101.6 Bmi: 18.9 Body Fat: 21.0

28.07.2011
Weight: 101.2 Bmi: 18.8 Body Fat: 20.8

26.07.2011
Weight: 102.0 Bmi: 19.0 Body Fat: 21.1

23.07.2011
Weight: 102.4 Bmi: 19.0 Body Fat: 21.1

11.07.2011
Weight: 101.4 Bmi: 18.8 Body Fat: 20.8

10.07.2011
Weight: 102.6 Bmi: 19.1 Body Fat: 21.3

08.07.2011
Weight: 102.0 Bmi: 19.0 Body Fat: 21.1

06.07.2011
Weight: 101.4 Bmi: 18.8 Body Fat: 20.8

02.07.2011
Weight: 102.6 Bmi: 19.1 Body Fat: 21.3

28.06.2011

Even though my BMI started in the normal range of 19.1, I wanted to test and demonstrate my simple weight loss plan for you! So you can see that applying my easy and effortless weight loss education plan resulted in a loss of ½ a stone over 2 months! Anorexia is classified as a BMI of under 17.5, so I have now stopped applying the weight loss plan at a BMI of 17.8. I merely wished to demonstrate to you that anyone can lose weight with my easy cost-free plan and stop at any weight they so desire! I don't recommend you personally aim for a body mass index below 19 however.

So in summary 4 x 4 exercise = 4 hours x 4 times a week of walking = 1000 calories a day or 4,000 calories a week!

A pound of weight (lb) = 3,500 calories. So by adding walking to one's daily activities, one can lose a lb a week in weight!

Now add to this the simple food plan that asks you to think twice between two choices of filling meals which only differ in calorie content. Go for the 200-300 'I can't believe it's only' calorie meal and not the 800-900 'extra hidden' calorie meal. This then adds another 500 calories a day of weight loss or over a week, 3,500 calories or one lb of weight loss! So in addition to the easy walking exercise, by choosing the tummy-filling but lower calorie meal, you lose yet another lb of weight each week without ever going hungry or skipping meals!

When you also apply the drink only water, freshly squeezed orange juice, and the occasional tea or coffee, if you must advice, you see that you have reduced your weekly intake of sugary coca cola (2 cans a day or 300 calories a day) and pints of beer (4 pints at 200 calories a pint) = 2100 'extra hidden' calories of coca cola + 800 'empty' calories of beer by 2,900 calories a week. Take off another lb of weight a week without even breaking out a sweat or starving!

The final chapter talks about maintenance. Now that you have reached your desired goal, how do we maintain this ideal goal weight forever?!

CHAPTER ELEVEN: MAINTENANCE

The second hardest part about 'dieting' is keeping the weight off. This is because the 'diet' is a deviation from your normal lifestyle. When the 'weight loss programme' becomes incorporated into your everyday lifestyle, it becomes habit-forming.

Once your palate has become accustomed to fried rice without the heavy sauces or grilled or broiled chicken without the curry sauce, you will start craving your healthier options.

If you change your normal routine by going on holiday, be mindful and do not book all-inclusive holidays with half or full board. What invariably happens on these cruises or fully-catered sun holidays, is that you break from your normal routine and stop thinking. You turn into a voracious creature who must eat twice as much as normal because a buffet is free! Believe me you will gain 10 lbs in one week without even blinking! Add to this the impulse to just bask by the pool at 36 calories an hour and one can see how quickly one's inactivity and over-eating can lead to gaining a stone in weight!

So to avoid this harsh temptation, book bed and breakfast holidays and make your own choices for lunch and dinner.

To work out how much walking and how many total calories you may consume in meals to maintain your ideal weight, I like to use the number 13.

If you stand 5'1" in height and wish to remain at a BMI of 20 (normal weight) using the BMI formula, you should maintain a weight of approximately 48 kilograms or

105 lbs or 7 ½ stone. So to maintain this weight of 105 lbs, multiply weight in lbs by 13 to get 1365 total daily calories.

As long as your daily activities total around 1365 calories, you cannot gain or lose weight; you remain static. Let's say you sleep for 8 hours. 8 x 36 calories an hour sleeping = 208 calories.

Let's say you spend 4 hours watching television in the evenings. 4 x 44 calories an hour of sitting and watching television = 176 calories.

Let's say you spend 8 hours a day sitting in meetings or at your desk. 8 x 96 calories an hour sitting in meetings = 768 calories.

We are now up to 1152 calories and have 4 hours left remaining in your 24-hour day to fill with activities. You have consumed 1365 calories so now have to expend 1365 – 1152 calories = 213 calories over the last 4 hours of your day or at least 53 calories an hour.

It means you have to do a bit more than sit in front of your computer (47 calories an hour) or watch television (44 calories an hour), so a bit of walking, house cleaning, gardening, house decluttering, playing with your children, walking the dog, window shopping, grocery shopping, travelling to/from work on the tube or British Rail, queueing in line at the post office, and so on and so forth, will easily fill up the remaining 4 hours and allow you to maintain your ideal weight for an eternity without even trying.

CHAPTER TWELVE:

10 REASONS NOT TO BE OBESE

1. Type II diabetes is more prevalent in obese middle-aged people with a BMI over 30. Diabetes is the leading cause of blindness and the 7th leading cause of death. 71,382 death certificates in the United States listed diabetes as the cause of death in 2007. Once you are diagnosed with diabetes, there is no turning back.

2. Obesity puts you at risk of cancer of the breast, cervix, colon, gallbladder, ovaries and uterus (womb). Excess adipose (fat) cells are carcinogenic, i.e. cause cancer.

3. Obesity puts added pressure and strain on your joints and leads to premature osteoarthritis of the lower back, hips and knees.

4. Obese people often suffer from obstructive sleep apnoea and stop breathing at night. Not to mention the loud snoring that disrupts any relationship!

5. Obesity puts one at risk of heart disease and stroke, the leading causes of premature death! Very high fatty content of cholesterol in your blood makes your arteries sticky and more vulnerable to plaque/clot formation that may block your heart or brain vessels.

6. Gallstones are more prevalent in obese people.

7. Society unfairly discriminates against obese people both socially and in the work place.

8. Obesity can lead to morbid obesity and being wheel-chair and/or home bed-bound. Fungal infections may occur in the skin folds and creases. Bed sores can occur if lying in one position for long periods of time.

9. Obesity prevents you from enjoying what normal people enjoy…shopping, travelling on public transportation, playing with your children, etc.

10. Premature death. Obesity shortens your life expectancy by at least 10 years.

I hope this book will help you, the reader, understand about weight gain and weight loss. It is a simple concept and something that can be fixed if you have the balance wrong. If this book turns around just one person's life and saves one life from an early grave, I am happy. I was too late to reach my close working colleague. I have often felt as though I wanted to spend an entire day with any obese person to show them how easy it is to lose weight, as I have done with each contributor on the Turn Back Your Body Clock television series and with this book, using myself as a guinea pig! You can do it too! Turn your life around and add at least 10 years longer to your life and well-being!

Other book titles by Dr Una Coales available from www.lulu.com.

Dr Una Coales's MRCGP AKT Hot Topic. RRP £29.99.
ISBN 978-1-4461-5675-9.

Dr Una Coales's MRCGP CSA Book. RRP £26.99.
ISBN 978-1-4461-5487-8.

How to find a husband, preferably a millionaire. RRP £12.99.
ISBN 978-1-4461-5964-4.